Yin Yoga for Beginners

Understanding the Importance of Yin Yoga

By

Cael Duthac

Table of Contents

CHAPTER 1

Introduction

1.1 What is Yin Yoga

Yin Yoga is a distinct and deeply meditative style of yoga that differs significantly from the more popular and dynamic forms of yoga, such as Vinyasa or Hatha. Developed in the late 1970s by Paulie Zink and later popularized by Paul Grilley and Sarah Powers, Yin Yoga focuses on the passive and static stretching of connective tissues, primarily targeting the fascia, ligaments, and tendons rather than the muscles. This approach stands in contrast to the more dynamic and muscle-centric practices that dominate Western yoga traditions.

Yin Yoga gets its name from the ancient Chinese philosophy of Yin and Yang, which represents opposing and complementary forces in the universe. In this context, Yin represents the passive, receptive, and cool aspects, while Yang symbolizes the active, dynamic, and warm aspects. Yin Yoga, therefore, embodies the Yin qualities by encouraging practitioners to hold poses for an extended period (usually three to five minutes or even longer), promoting stillness, and emphasizing surrender to gravity.

Yin poses are typically seated or lying down, and they aim to create gentle stress on the connective tissues. This stress stimulates the tissues to gradually release and lengthen, promoting improved joint mobility and overall flexibility. Yin Yoga is also deeply intertwined with mindfulness and meditation practices, making it a holistic approach to physical and mental well-being.

1.2 Benefits of Yin Yoga

The practice of Yin Yoga offers a multitude of benefits, both physical and mental, making it a valuable addition to one's wellness routine. Here are some of the key advantages:

Improved Flexibility: Yin Yoga targets the connective tissues, helping to increase joint mobility and flexibility. Over time, regular practice can lead to greater range of motion and reduced stiffness in the body.

Enhanced Body Awareness: The long holds and meditative nature of Yin Yoga encourage practitioners to develop a heightened sense of body awareness. This mindfulness can extend beyond the mat, leading to improved posture and body mechanics in daily life.

Stress Reduction: The emphasis on stillness and deep breathing in Yin Yoga promotes relaxation and stress reduction. It activates the parasympathetic nervous system, which counteracts the "fight or flight" response and induces a state of calm and balance.

Mental Clarity: The meditative aspect of Yin Yoga helps quiet the mind and improve concentration. Regular practice can lead to greater mental clarity and an increased ability to manage stress and emotional challenges.

Balancing Energy: Yin Yoga is often associated with the meridian system of Traditional Chinese Medicine. By targeting specific meridians in poses, it is believed to promote the balanced flow of energy (or "Qi") throughout the body, which can contribute to overall well-being.

Injury Prevention: By gently stretching and strengthening the connective tissues, Yin Yoga can help reduce the risk of injuries, particularly in areas prone to tightness and stiffness, such as the lower back and hips.

Holistic Healing: Some practitioners turn to Yin Yoga as a complementary therapy for certain health conditions, such as chronic pain, anxiety, and insomnia. While not a substitute for medical treatment, it can provide relief and support for these conditions.

Yin Yoga offers a unique approach to yoga practice that emphasizes stillness, deep stretching, and mindfulness. Its benefits extend beyond physical flexibility to encompass mental and emotional well-being, making it a valuable tool for those seeking a balanced and holistic approach to health and self-care. As we explore this practice further in this guide, you'll discover how to incorporate Yin Yoga into your life and experience its transformative effects.

CHAPTER 2

Getting Started

2.1 Setting the Right Environment

Creating the right environment for your Yin Yoga practice is essential for a fulfilling and calming experience. Here's how to set the stage:

Space: Find a quiet and clutter-free space where you won't be disturbed during your practice. Ideally, this space should be peaceful and free from distractions. You might consider setting up a dedicated yoga corner or using a room with soft lighting.

Temperature: Yin Yoga is best practiced in a comfortably warm environment. A temperature range of 70-75 degrees Fahrenheit (21-24 degrees Celsius) is generally suitable. You can adjust this based on your personal preferences, but ensure it's warm enough to avoid discomfort during long holds.

Lighting: Soft and dim lighting can create a calming atmosphere. Consider using candles, incense, or soft lamps to set the right mood. Natural light is also a great option if you're practicing during the day.

2.2 Necessary Equipment

Yin Yoga doesn't require a lot of equipment, but a few items can enhance your practice:

Yoga Mat: While not strictly necessary, a yoga mat provides a comfortable and non-slip surface for your practice. Choose a mat that suits your preferences in terms of thickness and texture.

Props: Props like yoga blocks, bolsters, and blankets can be invaluable for supporting your body in various poses. They help you maintain proper alignment and make the poses more accessible, especially for beginners.

Meditation Cushion or Pillow: If you plan to incorporate meditation into your Yin Yoga practice, a cushion or pillow can provide comfort during seated meditation.

Timer or Stopwatch: Since Yin Yoga poses are held for an extended period, having a timer or stopwatch can help you keep track of your holds. You can use your smartphone or a dedicated timer.

2.3 Clothing and Comfort

Comfort is key in Yin Yoga, so choose clothing that allows for ease of movement and doesn't restrict your range of motion. Here's what to consider:

Clothing: opt for comfortable, breathable clothing that allows you to stretch and move freely. Avoid clothing with zippers, buttons, or anything that might dig into your skin during poses.

Layers: Yin Yoga involves long holds, which can lead to changes in body temperature. Layering your clothing allows you to adjust as needed to stay comfortable.

Bare Feet: Yin Yoga is typically practiced without shoes or socks to provide a better connection with the mat and a sense of grounding.

Accessories: You may also want to have a blanket or shawl nearby to cover yourself during the final relaxation (Savasana) to stay warm and comfortable.

Creating a suitable environment and gathering the necessary equipment and clothing, you'll be well-prepared to embark on your Yin Yoga journey with comfort and focus.

CHAPTER 3

Yin Yoga Basics

3.1 Understanding Yin and Yang

Yin Yoga draws its inspiration from the ancient Chinese philosophy of Yin and Yang. Understanding these concepts is crucial to appreciating the essence of Yin Yoga:

Yin and Yang Defined: Yin and Yang represent opposing yet interconnected forces in the universe. Yin is passive, receptive, cooling, and associated with qualities like stillness, darkness, and the moon. Yang is active, dynamic, heating, and linked to qualities like movement, brightness, and the sun.

Balance and Harmony: In Chinese philosophy, health and harmony are achieved when there is a balance between Yin and Yang energies within the body. An imbalance can lead to physical or emotional disharmony.

Application to Yin Yoga: In Yin Yoga, poses are designed to target the Yin aspects of the body, specifically the connective tissues, which are denser and less elastic than muscles. The long, passive holds in Yin Yoga poses allow practitioners to delve into the Yin aspect of their bodies, fostering balance and holistic well-being.

3.2 Principles of Yin Yoga

Yin Yoga is guided by several key principles that differentiate it from other yoga styles:

Long Holds: Poses in Yin Yoga are held for an extended duration, typically ranging from three to five minutes or even longer. This extended time frame allows for a deeper stretch and targets the connective tissues.

Stillness: Unlike more dynamic yoga styles that involve constant movement, Yin Yoga encourages stillness in poses. This stillness helps practitioners explore their physical and mental sensations, promoting mindfulness and inner reflection.

Gentle Stress: Yin Yoga poses apply gentle stress to the connective tissues. The intention is not to force the body into extreme stretches but rather to find the "edge," the point at which you feel a mild, comfortable sensation of stretch.

Mindfulness: Yin Yoga is as much a mental practice as it is a physical one. Practitioners are encouraged to observe their thoughts, emotions, and bodily sensations while holding poses, fostering self-awareness and relaxation.

Prop Usage: Props such as bolsters, blocks, and blankets are often used in Yin Yoga to support the body in poses, helping practitioners find a comfortable and sustainable position for extended holds.

3.3 Yin Yoga vs. Other Yoga Styles

Yin Yoga stands out among the various yoga styles due to its unique approach:

Yin vs. Yang Yoga: While Yin Yoga focuses on long holds and passive stretches, Yang styles like Vinyasa and Power Yoga emphasize dynamic movement and muscular engagement. Both Yin and Yang practices complement each other, providing a well-rounded yoga experience.

Physical vs. Energetic Focus: Many traditional yoga styles emphasize physical strength and flexibility. In contrast, Yin Yoga prioritizes the energetic and emotional aspects of yoga by working with the body's subtle energy and encouraging mindfulness.

Individualized Practice: Yin Yoga is highly adaptable and suitable for practitioners of all ages and fitness levels. It provides an opportunity for each person to explore their unique physical and mental boundaries.

As you delve further into your Yin Yoga practice, these foundational principles will guide you in your journey towards increased flexibility, mindfulness, and inner balance.

CHAPTER 4

Essential Yin Yoga Poses

4.1 Butterfly Pose (Baddha Konasana)

- **Pose Description:** Butterfly Pose, also known as Baddha Konasana, involves sitting with your spine straight and the soles of your feet together, allowing your knees to drop out to the sides. You can hold onto your feet or ankles and gently fold forward from your hips.

- **Target Areas:** Butterfly Pose primarily targets the inner thighs, groin, and lower back. It's an excellent pose for opening the hips and releasing tension in the lower spine.

- **Benefits:**

  - **Hip Flexibility:** Regular practice of Butterfly Pose can improve hip flexibility and mobility, making it a valuable pose for those with tight hips.

  - **Lower Back Relief:** The gentle forward fold can alleviate lower back discomfort and promote relaxation in the lumbar region.

  - **Stimulates Digestion:** This pose can also aid digestion by massaging the abdominal organs when you fold forward.

4.2 Child's Pose (Balasana)

- **Pose Description:** Child's Pose, or Balasana, is a resting pose in which you kneel with your big toes touching and knees apart. Sit back on your heels and extend your arms forward on the mat, bringing your forehead to the ground.

- **Target Areas:** This pose primarily stretches the back, hips, and thighs. It's a gentle way to release tension in the spine.

- **Benefits:**

  - **Stress Reduction:** Balasana is often used as a restorative and calming pose that helps alleviate stress and anxiety.

  - **Back Relief:** It provides a gentle stretch to the lower back and can be comforting for those with back pain.

- **Improved Posture:** Regular practice of Child's Pose can help improve posture by increasing awareness of the spine's alignment.

4.3 Dragon Pose (Yin Side Lunge)

- **Pose Description:** Dragon Pose, also known as Yin Side Lunge, involves stepping one foot forward into a lunge while keeping the other leg extended straight behind you. The front knee is bent, and you can use props or support if needed to maintain balance. You can vary the angle and width of the stance to target different areas of the hips.

- **Target Areas:** Dragon Pose stretches the hip flexors, groin, and hamstrings. It's an excellent pose for releasing tension in the hips and increasing flexibility.

- **Benefits:**

  - **Hip Flexor Release:** Dragon Pose can be particularly effective in releasing tension in the hip flexors, which can become tight due to prolonged sitting or physical activity.

  - **Improved Hip Mobility:** Regular practice can enhance hip mobility and reduce discomfort associated with tight hips.

- **Mind-Body Connection:** The pose requires focus and concentration, fostering a strong mind-body connection and promoting mindfulness.

Incorporating these essential Yin Yoga poses into your practice can help you improve flexibility, release tension, and experience the soothing and meditative aspects of Yin Yoga. As you explore these poses, remember to practice patience, mindfulness, and breath awareness, which are core principles of Yin Yoga.

4.4 Sphinx Pose (Salamba Bhujangasana)

- **Pose Description:** Sphinx Pose, also known as Salamba

Bhujangasana, is a gentle backbend that involves lying on your stomach with your legs extended and your elbows under your shoulders, forearms flat on the mat. The chest lifts slightly off the ground, and the gaze is forward or slightly upward.

- **Target Areas:** Sphinx Pose primarily stretches the lower back, spine, and chest. It's a gentle backbend suitable for beginners.

- **Benefits:**

  - **Spinal Flexibility:** Sphinx Pose helps improve spinal flexibility by gently arching the back.

- **Stress Relief:** It can alleviate tension in the lower back and promote relaxation.

- **Heart Opening:** The pose opens the chest and encourages a sense of expansiveness, both physically and emotionally.

4.5 Savasana (Corpse Pose)

- **Pose Description:** Savasana, often referred to as Corpse Pose, is a relaxation and meditation pose. It involves lying on your back with your legs extended and your arms resting comfortably at your sides.

The palms can be facing up, and you close your eyes.

- **Target Areas:** While Savasana doesn't target specific muscles or joints, it's a pose for deep relaxation and mental stillness.

- **Benefits:**

  - **Total Relaxation:** Savasana is the ultimate relaxation pose, allowing the body and mind to completely let go of tension and stress.

  - **Stress Reduction:** It's highly effective for reducing stress, anxiety, and promoting mental clarity.

  - **Integration:** Savasana allows you to integrate the benefits of your Yin Yoga practice, both physically and mentally, before concluding your session.

While Savasana is traditionally practiced at the end of a yoga session, it's essential to remember that it's a vital part of Yin Yoga practice too. It's an opportunity to absorb the benefits of the previous poses and foster a deep sense of relaxation.

Incorporating Sphinx Pose and Savasana into your Yin Yoga routine provides a balanced experience that includes gentle back bending and deep relaxation. As you practice these poses, focus on your breath and the sensations in your body, allowing them to guide you toward a sense of inner calm and stillness.

CHAPTER 5

Proper Yin Yoga Techniques

5.1 Breath Awareness

Breath awareness is a foundational technique in Yin Yoga, as it not only helps you stay present in each pose but also supports the release of tension and encourages relaxation. Here's how to cultivate breath awareness in your Yin Yoga practice:

Natural Breathing: In Yin Yoga, the breath should be natural and unforced. Unlike some other yoga styles where specific breath patterns are prescribed,

Yin Yoga encourages you to breathe naturally through your nose.

Observing the Breath: Begin each pose by taking a few moments to simply observe your breath. Pay attention to the rhythm, depth, and quality of your inhalations and exhalations. Notice any areas of tension or resistance in the body.

Deepening the Breath: As you settle into a Yin Yoga pose, aim to deepen your breath gradually. Inhale deeply through your nose, allowing your abdomen to expand as you fill your lungs. Exhale fully, releasing any tension or tightness in the body.

Maintaining Consistency: Throughout the long holds in Yin Yoga, maintain a consistent and steady breath. This helps calm the nervous system and enhances your ability to surrender to the pose.

Using the Breath: Your breath can be a powerful tool for releasing physical and mental tension. With each exhalation, visualize tension and stress melting away. As you inhale, imagine fresh energy and relaxation flowing into the areas of your body that need it most.

Breath as a Guide: Pay close attention to your breath as a guide in finding your edge in each pose. If your breath becomes strained or shallow, it may be an indication that you've pushed too far into the pose. Back off slightly to find a more comfortable and sustainable position.

Breath and Mindfulness: Breath awareness is closely linked to mindfulness in Yin Yoga. As you focus on your breath, you also cultivate a mindful awareness of the sensations in your body and the thoughts in your mind. This combination of breath and mindfulness is key to the meditative aspect of Yin Yoga.

Breath awareness is a practice in itself. It may take time to develop a deep connection with your breath during Yin Yoga, so be patient and gentle with yourself. Over time, this technique will become more natural and supportive of your overall Yin Yoga experience, helping you find stillness, release, and inner peace in each pose.

5.2 Finding Your Edge

Finding your edge is a fundamental principle in Yin Yoga and is essential for practicing safely and effectively. Your edge is the point at which you feel a gentle, but not painful, sensation of stretch or tension in a Yin Yoga pose. Here's a closer look at how to find your edge in Yin Yoga:

1. Start Gently: When you first move into a Yin Yoga pose, begin with a gentle approach. Don't push yourself too deep into the pose right away.

2. Pay Attention to Sensations: As you settle into the pose, pay close attention to the sensations in your body. Notice where you feel the stretch or tension. It might be in your muscles, connective tissues, or joints.

3. Use Your Breath: Your breath is a valuable tool for finding your edge. As you inhale, consciously relax and soften into the pose. As you exhale, explore the stretch by gently moving a fraction deeper if it feels comfortable.

4. Be Mindful of Pain: Yin Yoga is not about pushing into pain. If you feel sharp, shooting, or intense pain in a pose, you've gone too far. Pain is a signal from your body to back off. Always practice within your comfort zone to avoid injury.

5. Find Stillness: Once you've found your edge, aim to stay still in the pose. Yin Yoga is about holding poses for an extended period, so avoid fidgeting or readjusting too frequently.

6. Use Props: Props such as bolsters, blankets, and blocks can be incredibly helpful in finding your edge. They provide support and allow you to customize the pose to your body's needs.

7. Stay Patient: Your edge may evolve during the hold as your body begins to relax. Be patient and allow this natural progression to occur. Avoid forcing the stretch.

8. Mindful Exploration: As you hold the pose, continue to breathe deeply and mindfully explore your edge. You may notice that the sensation changes or diminishes over time. This is a sign that your body is adapting to the stretch.

9. Respect Your Limits: Yin Yoga is not a competition with yourself or others. Everyone's edge is different, and it can vary from day to day. Respect your body's limitations and practice self-compassion.

10. Use Props Liberally: Props can be your best friend in Yin Yoga. They can provide the necessary support to find your edge comfortably. Don't hesitate to use them to enhance your practice.

11. Listen to Your Body: Ultimately, your body knows best. It will communicate its boundaries and needs. Listen to these signals and honor them. Your edge should always be a place of mild, sustainable discomfort, never pain or strain.

Finding your edge in Yin Yoga is a dynamic and intuitive process. It requires tuning into your body, being patient, and practicing mindfulness. With time and practice, you'll become more attuned to your own limits and be able to find your edge in each pose, allowing you to experience the full benefits of Yin Yoga safely and effectively.

5.3 Holding Poses and Relaxation

Holding poses and relaxation are central elements of Yin Yoga that contribute to its unique benefits. Let's explore these aspects in more detail:

1. Prolonged Holds: In Yin Yoga, poses are typically held for an extended period, often ranging from three to five minutes or even longer. This extended duration allows you to go beyond the superficial layers of the muscles and access the deeper connective tissues, such as the fascia, ligaments, and tendons. It's during these prolonged holds that you can experience profound physical and mental release.

2. Surrender to Gravity: Yin Yoga encourages practitioners to surrender to gravity and let go of muscular effort. Unlike more dynamic yoga styles, Yin poses are passive in nature. Once you find your edge, relax your muscles and let the weight of your body gradually deepen the stretch. This approach helps release chronic tension and promotes relaxation.

3. Stillness and Mindfulness:

Holding poses for an extended duration fosters stillness and mindfulness. As you settle into a pose, you have the opportunity to observe physical sensations, thoughts, and emotions that arise. This mindful awareness is a key component of the practice, allowing you to connect with the present moment and cultivate a sense of inner peace.

4. Resistance to the Urge to Fidget:

It's common to experience discomfort or restlessness during Yin Yoga poses, especially as you explore your edge. However, resist the urge to fidget or adjust too frequently. Instead, use your breath and mental focus to find ease within the discomfort. This resistance to restlessness can be a valuable practice in itself, teaching you patience and mental resilience.

5. Props for Support: Props like bolsters, blankets, and blocks are often used in Yin Yoga to provide support and enhance relaxation. Props can make it more comfortable to hold poses for extended periods and help you find relaxation within the stretch.

6. Transitioning Mindfully: When transitioning between poses, do so mindfully and with awareness. Pay attention to how your body feels as you come out of a pose, and take your time moving into the next one. This

transition period can be an
opportunity for reflection and
deepening your mindfulness practice.

7. Final Relaxation (Savasana):
After completing your Yin Yoga
sequence, it's customary to finish with
Savasana, also known as Corpse Pose.
This pose allows you to integrate the
benefits of your practice, both
physically and mentally. In Savasana,
you fully relax your body, release any
residual tension, and allow the
benefits of your practice to settle in.

8. Benefits of Relaxation: The
combination of prolonged holds and
relaxation in Yin Yoga contributes to
several benefits, including increased
flexibility, improved joint health,
reduced stress, enhanced mental
clarity, and a sense of emotional
release. It's a practice that nurtures the
body and mind holistically.

Holding poses and relaxation are at the heart of Yin Yoga's therapeutic qualities. By embracing stillness, surrendering to gravity, and practicing mindfulness, you can experience profound physical and mental transformations through this practice. Over time, you'll find that Yin Yoga not only enhances your physical flexibility but also deepens your connection with yourself and promotes a lasting sense of well-being.

5.4 Modifications and Props

Modifications and the use of props play a significant role in Yin Yoga, enhancing your practice by making poses more accessible, comfortable, and safe. Here's how to incorporate modifications and props effectively:

1. Props for Support: Props such as bolsters, blankets, blocks, and cushions can be your allies in Yin Yoga. They provide support, promote relaxation, and help you find your edge comfortably.

2. Bolsters: Bolsters are large, firm cushions that are often used to support the body in various poses. They can be placed under your chest, hips, or knees to create elevation and reduce the intensity of a stretch.

3. Blankets: Blankets can be folded and placed under sensitive areas, such as the knees or ankles, to cushion and support. They also help regulate body temperature during longer holds.

4. Blocks: Yoga blocks can be used to raise the floor to meet you in certain poses. Placing blocks under your hands, forearms, or sit bones can help you find a comfortable and sustainable position.

5. Cushions and Pillows: Soft cushions or pillows can be used to make sitting or lying poses more comfortable. They can be particularly helpful if you have discomfort in your hips or lower back.

6. Straps: Straps can be used to extend your reach in certain poses. They allow you to gently pull or push on specific body parts to encourage a deeper stretch without strain.

7. Personalized Support: Experiment with different props and their placements to find what works best for your body in each pose. Everyone's anatomy is unique, so personalizing your prop usage can significantly enhance your experience.

8. Modifications for Comfort: In Yin Yoga, comfort is essential. If you find that a traditional pose is too intense or uncomfortable, consider modifying it. For example, if sitting cross-legged is challenging, you can sit on a cushion or use props to elevate your hips.

9. Prop Usage Throughout the Pose: Don't hesitate to adjust your props as needed during the hold. As your body relaxes and the sensation changes, you may find that you need more or less support.

10. Props for Relaxation: Props can enhance relaxation during the pose. For example, placing a blanket over your body in Savasana can provide warmth and a sense of security.

11. Gradual Reduction: Over time, you can experiment with reducing the use of props as your flexibility and comfort in poses improve. The goal is to find a balance between support and challenge that works for you.

12. Safety and Comfort: Always prioritize safety and comfort over aesthetics or achieving a particular shape in a pose. Yin Yoga is about feeling the pose, not necessarily achieving an advanced variation.

incorporating modifications and props into your Yin Yoga practice, you can make poses more accessible and enjoyable. They enable you to find your edge with greater comfort, which ultimately enhances the benefits of the practice and reduces the risk of strain or injury. Props and modifications are tools to support your journey of self-discovery and deepening your practice.

CHAPTER 6

Creating a Yin Yoga Routine

6.1 Sample Yin Yoga Sequences

Creating a Yin Yoga routine involves selecting a sequence of poses that address your specific needs and goals. Here's another sample Yin Yoga sequence to inspire your practice. Remember, you can modify it based on your preferences and areas of focus:

Sample Yin Yoga Sequence #2

1. **Butterfly Pose (Baddha Konasana):** Begin with

Butterfly Pose to open the hips and groins.

2. **Child's Pose (Balasana):** Transition into Child's Pose for relaxation and lower back relief.

3. **Sphinx Pose (Salamba Bhujangasana):** Move into Sphinx Pose to gently stretch the chest and spine.

4. **Dragon Pose (Yin Side Lunge):** Embrace Dragon Pose to open the hip flexors and groin.

5. **Banana Pose:** Transition to Banana Pose for a side stretch.

6. **Saddle Pose (Supta Virasana with Props):** Open the chest and thighs with Saddle Pose, supported by props.

7. **Twisted Roots Pose:** Release tension in the spine with Twisted Roots Pose.

8. **Reclining Twist:** Lie on your back and bring one knee toward your chest, then guide it across your body for a gentle twist. Repeat on both sides.

9. **Wide-Knee Child's Pose:** Sit on your heels with knees wide apart and fold forward for a gentle hip opener.

10. **Savasana (Corpse Pose):** Conclude your practice with Savasana for deep relaxation.

6.2 Duration and Frequency

- **Duration:** In Yin Yoga, aim to hold each pose for a minimum of 3-5 minutes or longer if comfortable. Over time, you can gradually increase the duration as your flexibility and comfort in the poses improve.

- **Frequency:** You can practice Yin Yoga 2-3 times a week to start. As you become more experienced, you might choose to incorporate it into your daily routine or combine it with other yoga styles. Consistency is key for experiencing the full benefits of Yin Yoga.

6.3 Listening to Your Body

Listening to your body is a fundamental principle in Yin Yoga. Here's why it's essential:

- **Awareness:** Pay attention to how your body feels during each pose. Notice sensations, tension, or discomfort. Your body communicates its needs and limits through these sensations.

- **Adjustments:** Be willing to make adjustments as needed. If a pose feels too intense, use props, modify the pose, or come out of it altogether. Your comfort and safety are top priorities.

- **Mindfulness:** Cultivate mindfulness throughout your practice. Observe your breath, thoughts, and emotions without judgment. This awareness helps you make informed choices during your practice.

- **Variations:** Remember that your body is unique, and your edge may vary from day to day. Don't compare yourself to others. Respect your body's limitations, and celebrate your progress, no matter how small.

- **Rest When Necessary:** Yin Yoga encourages stillness, but if you ever feel the need to rest in a comfortable position (e.g., Child's Pose or Savasana) between poses, do so. Rest is an essential part of the practice.

- **Consistency:** Consistency in your practice allows you to develop a deeper understanding of your body and its needs. Over time, you'll become more attuned to your edges and find greater ease in your practice.

Yin Yoga is a journey of self-discovery and inner exploration. By creating a balanced routine, practicing regularly, and tuning into your body's signals, you'll develop a fulfilling Yin Yoga practice that supports your physical, mental, and emotional well-being. Remember that Yin Yoga is a practice of patience, acceptance, and self-compassion, so enjoy the process and the benefits it brings.

CHAPTER 7

Yin Yoga for Mindfulness

Yin Yoga is a powerful practice for cultivating mindfulness and meditation. It encourages a deep connection between the body, breath, and mind, fostering a state of heightened awareness and presence. Let's explore meditation and mindfulness in Yin Yoga, as well as the benefits of a mindful Yin Yoga practice:

7.1 Meditation and Mindfulness in Yin Yoga

Meditation in Yin Yoga: Meditation is an integral part of Yin Yoga, although it's often a subtle and gentle form of meditation. Here's how meditation is incorporated into Yin Yoga:

- **Stillness:** The extended holds in Yin Yoga naturally lead to a state of stillness. This stillness provides an ideal environment for meditation, allowing you to focus inward and observe your thoughts and sensations.

- **Breath Awareness:** Yin Yoga emphasizes breath awareness. As you hold poses, you pay close attention to your breath, which serves as an anchor for your meditation practice. This breath-centered meditation enhances your ability to stay present.

- **Observation:** Yin Yoga encourages you to observe physical sensations, thoughts, and emotions as they arise. This observational awareness is a form of meditation that promotes mindfulness.

Mindfulness in Yin Yoga:
Mindfulness is a core aspect of Yin Yoga, and it's interwoven throughout the practice:

- **Present Moment Awareness:** Yin Yoga invites you to be fully present in the moment. You observe the sensations in your body, the quality of your breath, and the thoughts that pass through your mind without judgment.

- **Acceptance:** Mindfulness in Yin Yoga involves accepting whatever arises in your experience, whether it's discomfort in a pose or distractions in your mind. It's about acknowledging what is without resistance.

- **Non-Judgment:** There's no judgment in Yin Yoga. You accept your body's limitations and meet yourself where you are in each pose. This non-judgmental attitude fosters self-compassion.

- **Breath and Body Connection:** Mindfulness in Yin Yoga is also about connecting with your body through your breath. You use your breath to explore sensations, release tension, and create a sense of ease within discomfort.

7.2 Benefits of Mindful Yin Yoga Practice

A mindful Yin Yoga practice offers a range of physical, mental, and emotional benefits:

- **Stress Reduction:** Mindfulness in Yin Yoga helps reduce stress by calming the nervous system and promoting relaxation. You learn to respond to stressors with equanimity.

- **Improved Flexibility:** Mindful stretching in Yin Yoga gradually improves flexibility and mobility in the joints, muscles, and connective tissues.

- **Enhanced Self-Awareness:** Through mindfulness, you gain a deeper understanding of your body and mind. This self-awareness extends beyond your mat and into your daily life.

- **Emotional Regulation:** Mindful Yin Yoga can assist in emotional regulation by providing a safe space to observe and process emotions that arise during practice.

- **Improved Concentration:** The meditative aspect of Yin Yoga enhances your ability to concentrate and stay focused, both on and off the mat.

- **Enhanced Mind-Body Connection:** Mindfulness

strengthens the mind-body
connection, allowing you to
listen to your body's signals and
respond to them appropriately.

- **Inner Peace:** Over time, a
  mindful Yin Yoga practice can
  lead to a deep sense of inner
  peace, contentment, and a
  reduction in mental chatter.

- **Resilience:** Mindfulness
  cultivates resilience by teaching
  you to accept discomfort and
  challenges with grace and
  poise.

Incorporating mindfulness into your
Yin Yoga practice can transform it
into a profound journey of self-
discovery and inner exploration. It
offers a pathway to greater self-
acceptance, emotional balance, and a
deeper connection with the present

moment. Over time, you'll find that the benefits of a mindful Yin Yoga practice extend far beyond your mat and into all aspects of your life.

CHAPTER 8

Yin Yoga and Your Well-being

Yin Yoga is a holistic practice that offers a wide range of physical, mental, and energetic benefits to support your overall well-being. Let's explore some of these benefits in more detail:

8.1 Stress Reduction and Relaxation

Yin Yoga is particularly effective for stress reduction and relaxation. Here's why:

- **Calms the Nervous System:** The extended holds in Yin Yoga activate the parasympathetic nervous system, which is responsible for the "rest and digest" response. This promotes a sense of calm and relaxation, reducing stress and anxiety.

- **Release of Tension:** The long holds in Yin poses encourage the release of physical tension and tightness in the body. This physical release often parallels a mental and emotional release, creating a profound sense of relaxation.

- **Mindfulness and Presence:** Yin Yoga cultivates mindfulness and present-moment awareness. By focusing on the sensations in your body and your breath, you become fully immersed in the practice, letting go of worries and distractions.

- **Stress Resilience:** Regular practice of Yin Yoga can enhance your ability to respond to stressors in a more composed and resilient manner. It provides a toolbox of relaxation techniques that you can use in daily life.

8.2 Improved Flexibility and Joint Health

Yin Yoga is excellent for improving flexibility and promoting joint health:

- **Deep Stretch:** The prolonged holds allow for a deep, sustained stretch in muscles and connective tissues. This gradually improves flexibility, especially in areas like the hips, pelvis, and lower back.

- **Joint Mobility:** Yin Yoga targets the joints and helps maintain or improve their range of motion. It's particularly beneficial for joint health as it lubricates the joints and prevents stiffness.

- **Prevention of Injury:** Improved joint health and flexibility reduce the risk of injury in daily activities and other physical pursuits.

8.3 Balancing Energy Flow

Yin Yoga is rooted in traditional Chinese medicine principles of balancing the body's energy flow or Qi (pronounced "chee"). Here's how it helps balance energy:

- **Meridian Stimulation:** Yin Yoga poses often target specific meridians, which are energy pathways in the body according to traditional Chinese medicine. By stimulating these meridians, Yin Yoga helps balance the flow of energy.

- **Yin and Yang Balance:** Yin Yoga complements more dynamic forms of yoga and exercise, which are considered yang practices. Balancing yin and yang energies is believed to promote overall health and vitality.

- **Emotional and Energetic Release:** As you hold poses and release physical tension, you may also release emotional and energetic blockages. This can lead to a sense of emotional balance and harmony.

- **Mind-Body Connection:** Yin Yoga encourages a strong mind-body connection, allowing you to tune into the subtle sensations of energy in your body.

Incorporating Yin Yoga into your well-being routine can provide a profound sense of balance, relaxation, and vitality. Whether you're seeking stress reduction, increased flexibility, or a deeper connection with your body and energy, Yin Yoga offers a valuable path to support your overall well-being.

CHAPTER 9

Common Challenges and Solutions

Yin Yoga can be a deeply rewarding practice, but like any form of yoga, it comes with its own set of challenges. Here are some common challenges practitioners may face in Yin Yoga and practical solutions for each:

9.1 Physical Discomfort

Challenge: Yin Yoga poses can be uncomfortable, and it's common to experience physical discomfort during the extended holds. This discomfort may manifest as tightness, tension, or even mild pain.

Solution:

1. **Mindful Breathing:** Use your breath as a tool to manage discomfort. Take slow, deep breaths and consciously release tension with each exhale.

2. **Find Your Edge:** Experiment with finding the right level of intensity. Remember, Yin Yoga is about mild, sustainable discomfort, not pain. Adjust the pose or use props to find a more comfortable edge.

3. **Stay Present:** Focus on the sensations in your body rather than resisting them. Observing the discomfort without judgment can reduce its intensity.

4. **Use Props:** Props like bolsters, blankets, and blocks can provide support and make poses more comfortable. Don't hesitate to use them liberally.

5. **Acceptance:** Embrace the discomfort as an opportunity for growth. Over time, your body may adapt, and what was once uncomfortable may become more manageable.

9.2 Impatience and Restlessness

Challenge: Yin Yoga requires patience and stillness, which can be challenging for those accustomed to more active yoga styles or fast-paced lifestyles. Restlessness and impatience may arise during the long holds.

Solution:

1. **Set Realistic Expectations:** Understand that Yin Yoga is a slow-paced practice designed for introspection and relaxation. Adjust your expectations accordingly.

2. **Mindful Focus:** Redirect your mind to your breath and the sensations in your body whenever restlessness arises.

This can help anchor your attention and reduce mental agitation.

3. **Use Breath Awareness:** Pay close attention to your breath. Cultivate a steady and rhythmic breath pattern to calm the mind.

4. **Practice Patience:** Consider the restlessness as an opportunity to cultivate patience and mental resilience. View it as part of the practice itself.

5. **Gradual Progress:** Recognize that progress in Yin Yoga is often gradual. Over time, you may find it easier to remain still and patient.

9.3 Staying Consistent

Challenge: Maintaining a consistent Yin Yoga practice can be challenging due to busy schedules or a lack of motivation.

Solution:

1. **Schedule Regular Sessions:** Set aside dedicated time for Yin Yoga in your weekly schedule. Consistency is key, so treat it as a non-negotiable appointment with yourself.

2. **Shorter Sessions:** If time is limited, consider shorter Yin sessions. Even 10-15 minutes of practice can be beneficial.

3. **Combine with Yang Yoga:** Incorporate Yin sessions as a complement to your more dynamic yoga or exercise

routine. This can help you stay consistent while reaping the benefits of both styles.

4. **Accountability Partner:**
Practice with a friend or join a class to hold yourself accountable. Sharing the practice can also be motivating.

5. **Variety:** Explore different Yin Yoga sequences and poses to keep your practice interesting and engaging.

6. **Mindful Journaling:** Keep a Yin Yoga journal to track your progress and experiences. This can serve as a source of motivation and reflection.

Addressing these common challenges with mindfulness, patience, and adaptability, you can navigate your Yin Yoga practice more effectively and reap the numerous benefits it offers. Remember that Yin Yoga is a personal journey, and the challenges you encounter are opportunities for growth and self-discovery.

CHAPTER 10

Advanced Yin Yoga Practices

Advanced Yin Yoga practices build upon the foundational principles of

Yin Yoga but may incorporate more challenging elements. Here are two advanced aspects of Yin Yoga:

10.1 Longer Holds and Deeper Stretches

Challenge: Prolonged holds and deeper stretches in Yin Yoga require a deeper level of patience, flexibility, and mental focus. Advanced practitioners may seek to extend the duration of their holds or explore more intense sensations.

Solution:

1. **Progress Gradually:** If you wish to increase the duration of your holds or deepen your stretches, do so incrementally. Add 30 seconds to a minute to

your usual hold times, but do it mindfully.

2. **Maintain Breath Awareness:** Advanced Yin Yoga practices should still prioritize breath awareness. Focus on deep, steady breaths to support you during longer holds and deeper stretches.

3. **Use Props Wisely:** Even in advanced practices, props can be invaluable. They allow you to find your edge without pushing too far. Experiment with different props to enhance your practice.

4. **Prioritize Safety:** Always prioritize safety over achieving extreme sensations. Avoid pain or excessive discomfort. The goal is not to force your body

but to gently explore your limits.

10.2 Combining Yin Yoga with Other Practices

Challenge: Advanced Yin Yoga practitioners may seek to integrate Yin with other yoga styles or holistic practices to create a more comprehensive approach to well-being.

Solution:

1. **Yin-Yang Fusion:** Combine Yin Yoga with Yang Yoga styles like Vinyasa or Hatha for a balanced practice. Start with Yin to cultivate mindfulness and flexibility, then transition into a dynamic Yang practice for strength and vitality.

2. **Meditation Integration:**
   Advanced practitioners can
   deepen their practice by
   incorporating meditation before
   or after Yin Yoga sessions.
   This combination enhances
   mental clarity and self-
   awareness.

3. **Breathing Techniques:**
   Explore pranayama (breath
   control) techniques in
   conjunction with Yin Yoga.
   Breathwork can intensify the
   effects of Yin poses and
   promote energetic balance.

4. **Holistic Wellness:** Consider
   combining Yin Yoga with
   holistic practices such as
   mindfulness meditation,
   acupuncture, or traditional
   Chinese medicine for a holistic
   approach to well-being.

5. **Chakra Work:** Some advanced practitioners incorporate chakra balancing techniques into Yin Yoga. Specific poses and visualizations can target and balance individual chakras.

6. **Teacher Training:** If you're interested in advanced Yin Yoga practices, consider enrolling in a Yin Yoga teacher training program. These programs provide in-depth knowledge and advanced techniques.

When advancing your Yin Yoga practice, it's essential to maintain a mindful and balanced approach. Remember that safety and self-care should always come first. Advanced practices should be pursued with a solid foundation in Yin Yoga and a deep respect for your body's limits.

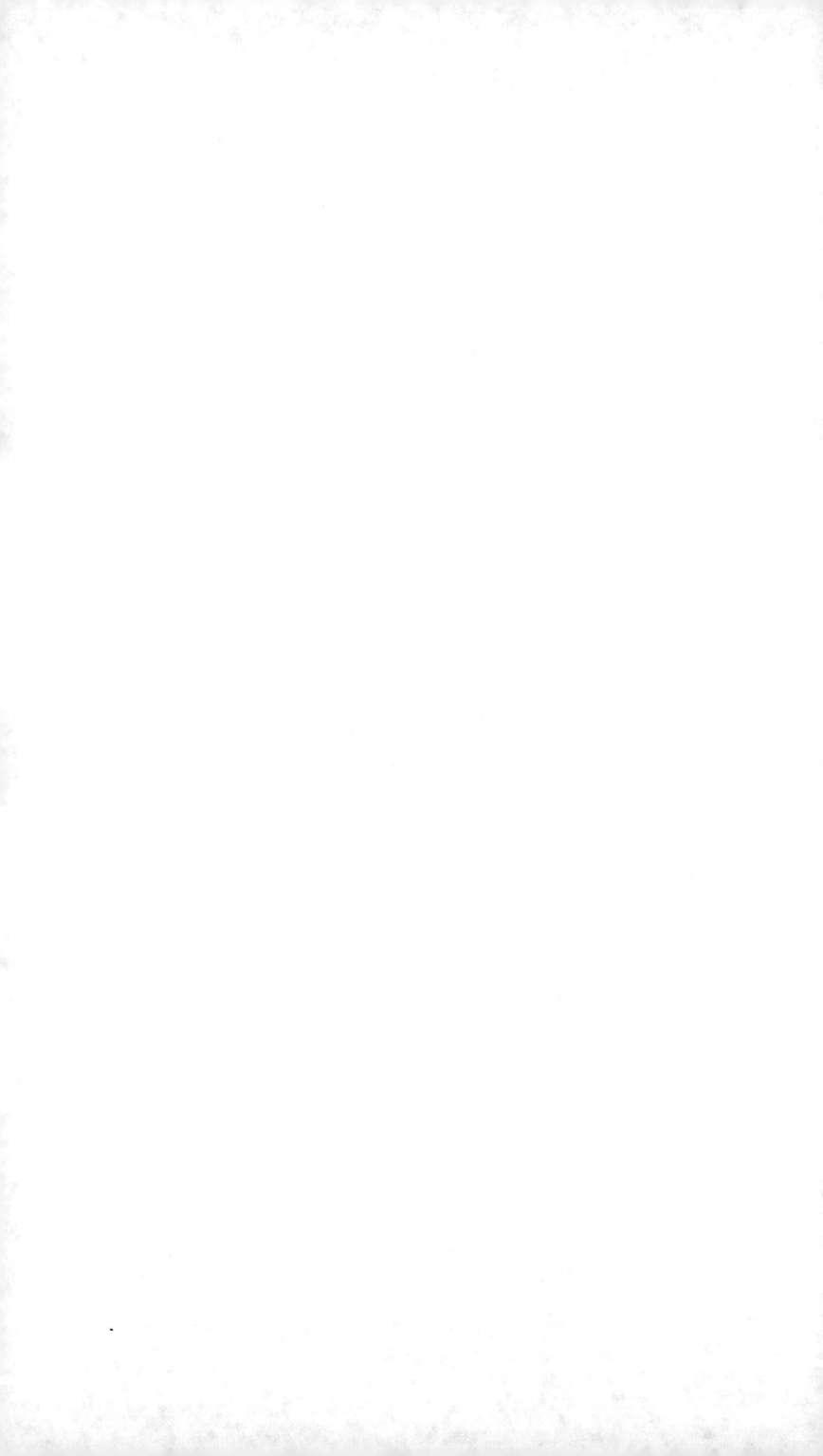

www.ingramcontent.com/pod-product-compliance
Lightning Source LLC
Chambersburg PA
CBHW062357290526
45794CB00005B/2267